CHAFFL

MW01232531

FOR KETOGENIC

DIET

LOSE WEIGHT BY STIMULATING THE BRAIN AND
METABOLISM: DELICIUS RECIPES LOW CARB TO
INTEGRATE YOUR KETOGENIC DIET

CHRISTINE BUCKLEY

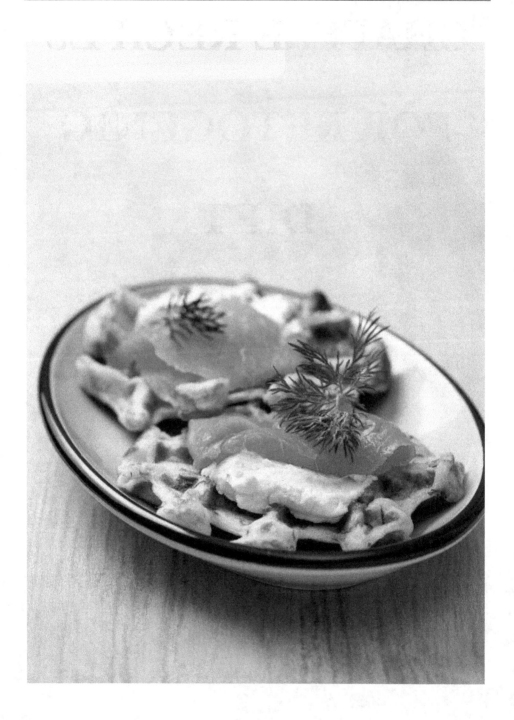

The information in the following pages is broadly considered a truthful and accurate account of facts and as such, any inattention, use, or misuse of the information in question by the reader will render any resulting actions solely under their purview. There are no scenarios in which the publisher or the original author of this work can be in any fashion deemed liable for any hardship or damages that may befall them after undertaking information described herein.

Additionally, the information in the following pages is intended only for informational purposes and should thus be thought of as universal. As befitting its nature, it is presented without assurance regarding its prolonged validity or interim quality. Trademarks that are mentioned are done without written consent and can in no way be considered an endorsement from the trademark holder.

TABLE OF CONTENTS

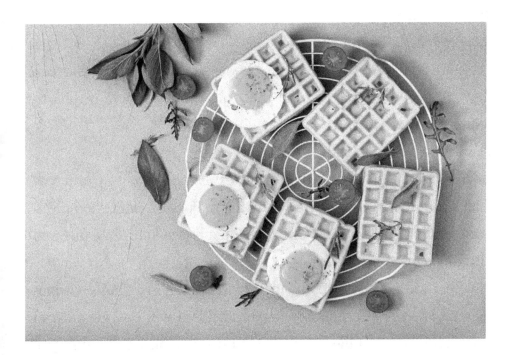

INTRODUCTION

Keto chaffles have taken the world by storm. Made with just two main ingredients, egg and butter, they can be prepared easily at home. You can eat them as sweet desserts, as a breakfast food, or as a snack. Chaffles are perfectly healthy foods that follow the

ketogenic diet recommendations.

They are high-fat, protein, and low-carbohydrate foods that can show the body how to use fat as an alternative source of fuel to produce energy and burn fat.

Thank you for downloading this book.

In this book, I will discuss chaffles and explain how they are different than waffles. I will ex- plain the various types of chaffles you can make easily at home. I will also go deep into the ketogenic diet and discuss its many advantages.

Finally, I will also share many mouth-watering Keto Chaffle recipes that are all easy to prepare. For each recipe, I will provide a list of ingredients and detailed step-by-step instructions. I am sure you will find this book very useful. Happy reading!

CHAPTER 1

FIRST OF ALL, WHAT IS A

CHAFFLE?

These "Chaffles" are nothing more than waffles made with cheese. Hence the name "Chaffle" which derives from the union "Cheese" + "Waf- fle". People tied to the keto diet usually love chaffles.

Grated cheese is a main ingredient in chaffle.

It's made with an egg and cheese batter instead of the flour-based batter you'll find in waffles. The high flour content in waffles adds a lot of carbohydrates, making them unhealthy according to the recommendations of the keto diet. Chaffles, on the other hand, have no flour. You can tell they're low-carb waffles with cheese.

The chaffles are extremely delicious. You won't realize that what you are actually eating is cheese eggs or cheese waffles. There are hundreds of chaffle recipes available, so you'll never miss out on options when you want to make one. There are also chaffles without cheese, for those who want to avoid or limit their intake of grated cheese.

CHAPTER 2

BENEFITS OF KETO DIET

The Keto diet has become so popular in recent years because of the success people have noticed. Not only have they lost weight, but scientific studies show that the Keto diet can help you improve your health in many others. As when starting any new diet or exercise routine, there may seem to be some disadvantages, so we will go over those for the Keto diet. But most people agree that the benefits outweigh the change period!

Benefits/Advantages

Losing weight: for most people, this is the foremost benefit of switching to Keto! Their previous diet method may have stalled for them, or they were noticing weight creeping back on. With Keto, studies have shown that people have been able to follow this diet and relay fewer hunger pangs and suppressed appetite while losing weight at the same time! You
are minimizing your carbohydrate intake, which means more occasional blood sugar spikes. Often, those fluctuations in
blood sugar levels make you feel hungrier and more prone to

snacking in between meals. Instead, by guiding the body towards ketosis, you are eating a more fulfilling diet of fat and protein and harnessing energy from ketone molecules instead of glucose. Studies show that low-carb diets effectively reduce visceral fat (the fat you commonly see around the abdomen increases as you become obese). This reduces your risk of obesity and improves your health in the long run.

Reduce the Risk of Type 2 Diabetes:

The problem with carbohydrates is how unstable they make blood sugar levels. This can be very dangerous for people who have diabetes or are pre-diabetic because of unbalanced blood sugar levels or family history. Keto is an excellent option because of the minimal intake of carbohydrates it requires. Instead, you are harnessing most of your calories from fat or protein, which will not cause blood sugar spikes and, ultimately, less pressured the pancreas to secrete insulin. Many studies have found that diabetes patients who followed the Keto diet lost more weight and eventually reduced their fasting glucose levels. This is monumental news for patients with unstable blood sugar levels or hopes to avoid or reduce their diabetes medication intake.

Improve cardiovascular risk symptoms to lower your chances of having heart disease:

Most people assume that following Keto is so high in fat content has to increase your risk of coronary heart disease or

heart attack. But the research proves otherwise! Research shows that switching to Keto can lower your blood pressure, increase your HDL good cholesterol, and reduce your triglyceride fatty acid levels.

That's because the fat you are consuming on Keto is healthy and high-quality fats, so they reverse many unhealthy symptoms of heart disease. They boost your "good" HDL cholesterol numbers and decrease your "bad" LDL cholesterol numbers. It also reduces the level of triglyceride fatty acids in the bloodstream. A top-level of these can lead to stroke, heart attack, or prema- ture death. And what are the top levels of fatty acids linked to?

High Consumption of Carbohydrates:

With the Keto diet, you are drastically cutting your intake of carbohydrates to improve fatty acid levels and improve other risk factors. A 2018 study on the Keto diet found that it can improve 22 out of 26 risk factors for cardiovascular heart disease! These factors can be critical to some people, especially those who have a history of heart disease in their family.

Increases the Body's Energy Levels:

Let's briefly compare the difference between the glucose molecules synthesized from a high carbohydrate intake versus
ketones produced on the Keto diet. The liver makes ketones
and use fat molecules you already stored.

This makes themmuch more energy-rich and an endless source of fuel compared to glucose, a simple sugar molecule. These ketones can give you a burst of energy physically and mentally, allowing you to have greater focus, clarity, and attention to detail.

Decreases inflammation in the body:

Inflammation on its own is a natural response by the body's immune system, but when it becomes uncontrollable, it can lead to an array of health problems, some severe and some minor. The health concerns include acne, autoimmune conditions, arthritis, psoriasis, irritable bowel syndrome, and even acne and eczema. Often, removing sugars and carbohydrates from your diet can help patients of these diseases avoid flare-ups - and the delightful news is Keto does just that! A 2008 research study found that Keto decreased a blood marker linked to high inflammation in the body by nearly 40%. This is glorious news for people who may suffer from inflammatory disease and want to change their diet to improve.

Increases your mental Functioning Level:

As we elaborated earlier, the energy-rich ketones can boost the body's physical and mental levels of alertness. Research has shown that Keto is a much better energy source for the brain than simple sugar glucose molecules are. With nearly 75% of your diet coming from healthy fats, the brain's neural cells and mitochondria have a better source of energy to function at the highest level. Some studies have tested patients on the Keto diet and found they had higher cognitive functioning, better memory recall, and were less susceptible to memory loss. The Keto diet can even decrease the occurrence of migraines, which can be very detrimental to patients.

Decreases risk of diseases like Alzheimer's, Parkinson's, and epilepsy.

They created the Keto diet in the 1920s to combat epilepsy in children. From there, research has found that Keto can improve your cognitive functioning level and protect brain cells from injury or damage. This is very good to reduce the risk of neurodegenerative disease, which begins in the brain

because of neural cells mutating and functioning with damaged parts or lower than peak optimal functioning.

Studies have found that the following Keto can improve the mental functioning of patients who suffer from diseases like Alzheimer's or Parkinson's. These neurodegenerative diseases

sadly, have no cure, but the Keto diet could improve symptoms as they progress. Researchers believe that it's because of cutting out carbs from your diet, which reduces the

occurrence of blood sugar spikes that the body's neural cells have to keep adjusting to.

Keto can regulate hormones in women who have PCOS (polycystic ovary syndrome) and PMS (pre-menstrual syn- drome).

Women who have PCOS suffer from infertility, which can be very heartbreaking for young couples trying to start a family. For this condition, there is no known cure, but we believe it's related to many similar diabetic symptoms like obesity and a high level of insulin. This causes the body to produce more sex hormones, which can lead to infertility. The Keto diet paved its way as a popular way to regulate insulin and hormone levels and increase a woman's chances of getting pregnant.

Disadvantages

Your body will have a Changed period: It depends from person to person on the number of days that will be, but when you start any new diet or exercise routine, your body has to adjust to the new normal. With the Keto diet, you are drastically cutting your carbohydrates intake, so the body must adjust to that. You may feel slow, weak, exhausted, and like you are not thinking as quick or fast as you used to. It just means that your body is adjusting Keto, and once this change period is done, you will see the weight loss results you expected.

If you are an athlete, you may need more carbohydrates:

If you still want to try Keto as an athlete, you must talk to your nutritionist or trainer to see how the diet can be tweaked for you. Most athletes require a greater intake of carbs than the Keto diet requires, which means they may have to up their intake to ensure they have the energy for their training sessions. High endurance sports (like rugby or soccer) and

heavy weightlifting requires more significant information on carbohy- drates. If you're an athlete wanting to follow Keto and gain the health benefits, it's crucial you first talk to your trainer before changing your diet.

You have to count your daily macros carefully:

For beginners, this can be tough, and even people already on Keto can become lazy about this. People are often used to eating what they want without worrying about just how many grams of protein or carbs it contains. With Keto, be meticulous about counting your intake to ensure you are maintaining the Keto breakdown (75% fat, 20% protein, ~5% carbs). The closer you stick to this, the better results you will see regard- ing weight loss and other health benefits. If your weight loss has stalled or you're not feeling as energetic as you hoped, it could be because your macros are off. Find a free calorie counting app that you look at the ingredients of everything you're eating and cooking.

CHAPTER 3

HOW TO MAKE THE PERFECT CHAFFLE

Here are some tips that will help you make fantastic chaffles

• Add a slice of chopped ham while mixing the egg and cheese. This will give you more protein and flavor. Those on a strict keto diet can also use bacon.

• Before adding the egg and cheese mixture, sprinkle some extra cheese on your waffle or chaffle maker. You will then have a savory and crispy chaffle.

• Don't open the waffle iron too early for checking. It should continue cooking until the chaffle is done and crisp. Let it cook for slightly longer for best results.

• Use mozzarella if you want your chaffle to be sweet. Cheddar cheese is good for savory chaffles. You can use Haloumi or goat cheese, but mozzarella is always the best

option because it is mild and not as greasy as many other

cheese varieties. Mozzarella will also reduce the eggy taste.

• Pepper jack cheese will give a slightly spicy taste. Almond/Coconut Flour in Chaffles

Chapter 4

SIMPLE CHAFFLE RECIPES

Mayonnaise & Cream Cheese Chaffles

Servings: 4 Cooking Time: 20 Minutes

Ingredients:

- 4 organic eggs large
- 4 tablespoons mayonnaise
- 1 tablespoon almond flour
- 2 tablespoons cream cheese, cut into small cubes

Directions:

Preheat a waffle iron and then grease it. In a bowl, place the eggs, mayonnaise and almond flour and with a hand mixer, mix until smooth. Place about ¼ of the mixture into preheated waffle iron.

Place about ¼ of the cream cheese cubes on top of the mixture evenly and cook for about 5 minutes or until golden brown.

Repeat with the remaining mixture and cream cheese cubes.
Serve warm.

Nutrition Info: Per Servings: Calories: 190 | Net Carb: 0.6g | Fat: 17g Saturated Fat: 4.2g | Carbohydrates: 0.8g | Dietary Fiber: 0.2g Sugar: 0.5g | Protein: 6.7g

Double Choco Chaffle

Servings: 2 Cooking Time: 10 Minutes

Ingredients:

- 1 egg
- 2 teaspoons coconut flour
- 2 tablespoons sweetener
- 1 tablespoon cocoa powder
- ¼ teaspoon baking powder
- 1 oz. cream cheese
- ½ teaspoon vanilla
- 1 tablespoon sugar-free chocolate chips

Directions:

Put all the ingredients in a large bowl. Mix well.

Pour half of the mixture into the waffle maker.
Seal the device.

Cook for 4 minutes.

Uncover and transfer to a plate to cool.

Repeat the procedure to make the second chaffle.

Nutrition Info:

Calories 171 | Total Fat 10.7g | Saturated Fat 5.3g | Cholesterol 97mg | Sodium 106mg | Potassium 179mg | Total Carbohydrate 3g | Dietary Fiber 4. | Protein 5.8g | Total Sugars 0.4g

Cheeseburger Chaffle

Servings: 2

Cooking Time: 15 Minutes

Ingredients:

- 1 lb. ground beef
- 1 onion, minced
- 1 tsp. parsley, chopped
- 1 egg, beaten
- Salt and pepper to taste
- 1 tablespoon olive oil
- 4 basic chaffles
- 2 lettuce leaves
- 2 cheese slices
- 1 tablespoon dill pickles
- Ketchup
- Mayonnaise

Directions:

In a large bowl, combine the ground beef, onion, parsley, egg, salt and pepper.

Mix well.

Form 2 thick patties. Add olive oil
to the pan.

Place the pan over medium heat.

Cook the patty for 3 to 5 minutes per side or until fully cooked. Place the patty on top of each chaffle.

Top with lettuce, cheese and pickles.

Squirt ketchup and mayo over the patty and veggies.
Top with another chaffle.

Nutrition Info: Calories 325Total Fat 16.3g Saturated Fat 6.5g Cholester- ol 157mg Sodium 208mg Total Carbohydrate 3g Dietary Fiber 0.7g Total Sugars 1.4g Protein 39.6g Potassium 532mg

Basic chaffle recipes

Here are four ways to create a basic chaffle. Chaffles work excellent as low carb keto bread, and they make fantastic low carb waffles, of course.

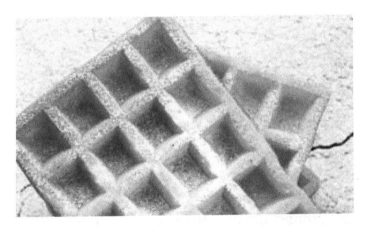

Servings: 1

Preparation time: 2 minutes

Nutritional values:

202 kcal Calories | 13 g Fat | 3 g
Carbs | 16 g Proteins

Ingredients

1 large egg

1/2 cup mozzarella cheese, finely grated

Directions

Preheat the waffle iron

Whisk up the one egg and the grated cheese with a fork in a tiny bowl unless mixed

Spread half of the mixture evenly well into the waffle

Cook for three or four minutes, or until golden brown. To cool, move onto a plate. Repeat the same for the remaining batter

Variations

Use 2 egg whites or a modest 1/4 cup of carton white eggs for an egg white chaffle. Divide as instructed and prepare.

Add 1/8 tsp maple extract to the egg / cheese mixture for a maple chaffle waffle.

Add 1 tbsp of finely ground almond flour to an almond waffle chaffle. Mix it well. Divide as instructed and prepare.

This recipe is for the friendliest degustation chaffles (with the exception of maple waffles). You can alter varieties with different cheeses, extracts and add-ins.

Other notes

Store in the refrigerator in an airtight jar for up to 3-4 days. Reheat toaster in a toaster oven. Freeze each of the chaffles individually in plastic wrap and place them in zip-top freezer bags. Store up to 3 months. Reheat-thaw in the refrigerator overnight, or softly thaw in the microwave at low power. Then toast in an oven or toaster to get the texture back.

Conquer Monsieur Or (Madame) Keto Chaffle Sandwich

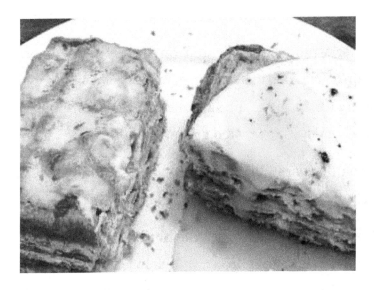

Servings: 1-2 Preparation time: 15 min

Ingredients

- 2 chaffles
- Gruyere cheese with thin slices (enough for 3 layers)
- 2 thinly sliced strips of ham (or one thicker slice)
- 1-2 tsp Dijon mustard (or to taste)
- 1 pack keto bechamel sauce

Directions

Make use of the chaffles with the crispy, savory chaffle instructions

The broiler would be preheated on maximum. Put one of the chaffles on a grill rack in a baking dish. Add a layer of gruyere sliced and add a layer of ham sliced. Pour Dijon mustard over the ham. Apply a second layer of grated gruyere over the ham and put the

second chaffle over it. Place the bechamel sauce over the top of the sandwich then place another sliced gruyere layer

Place the sandwich underneath the broiler before the cheese is melted, bubbly and light brown. Wait closely to guarantee it's not blackening Take away from the frying pan. Simply cover with a freshly baked, sun- ny side up fried egg, served with a touch of salt and pepper if creating it into a Croque madame. Top it with fresh parsley and enjoy

Nutritional Info:

360 kcal Calories | 18.4 g Fat | 9.5 g Carbs | 7.6 g Proteins

Keto Parmesan Garlic Chaffles – 3 Manner

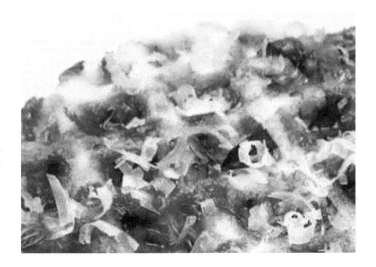

Servings: 2

Preparation Time: 2 minutes

Nutritional Values:

352 kcal Calories | 24 g Fat | 2 g
Carbs | 34 g Proteins

Ingredients

- 1/2 cup of mozzarella cheese, shredded
- 1 beaten egg
- 1/4 cup of Parmesan cheese, grated
- 1 tsp of Italian Seasoning
- 1/4 tsp of garlic powder

Directions

Switch on your mini Waffle Maker

Bring in all the products, with the exception of the mozzarella cheese, to a bowl and mix. Put in the cheese and blend till it's mixed well

Spray non-stick spray on your waffle plates then add half of the batter in the center. Shut the cover as well as cook for 3 to 5 min, depends entirely on how crisp you want in your chaffles

There are a few choices to serve. One is to represent with grated parme- san cheese, a drizzle of olive oil and chopped fresh parsley or basil NOTES

Transformations

• Italian chaffle sandwich
Start preparing the base recipe, as described above. Add lettuce and tomato, cold cuts and whatever you want to.

• Chaffle breadsticks
As mentioned above, make the base recipe. Slice each chaffle in 4 sticks then serve with sides of Marinara Sauce (low carb).

• Chaffle bruschetta
Start preparing the base mixture, as described above. Add 3 to 4 chopped cherry tomatoes, sliced, 1/2 tsp of chopped fresh basil and olive oil spray and a sprinkle of salt. Put over the upper part of the chaffles and serve as cooked above.

Keto Chaffle Pulled Pork Sandwich with Creamy Coleslaw

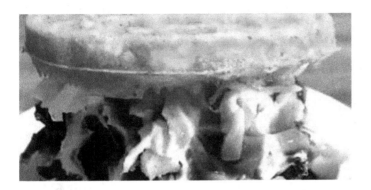

Servings: 4

Preparation time: 25 min.

Ingredients

- 1 pork butt - bone-in
- 8 tbsp barbecue sauce - free of sugar
- 1 packet of coleslaw mix or chopped cabbage
- 1 cup mayo
- 2 tbsp - heavy cream
- 1 tsp - creole mustard (any mustard you want, etc.)
- 1 tbsp erythritol. If you want a sweeter coleslaw, apply more erythritol (or any keto sugar substitute)
- 1 tsp (Optional) pepper
- 1 tsp garlic powder
- 1 tsp black chili pepper
- 1 tsp salt

Directions

Begins with "scoring" the roast's fat side. The scoring helps the seasoning to enter the fat and add this to another flavour

Use cooking oils, butter, mustard, Worcestershire sauce or any other chosen "wet" ingredient to add a slight element of moisture to enable the seasonings or rub to stick better to the meat

Cover the whole piece of meat absolutely with your favourite rub and let it sit for around 15-20 minutes until burning your Pit Barrel

Place the fat side of the pork butt on the grill so that the meat is covered, and the fat becomes crisper if you cut the pork into pieces for taste and texture pieces. Smoke exposed inside until it hits 165 degrees. Put it in a foil tray, cover it and position it again in the cooker once 205 degrees is achieved

Take out the pan and let it cool. To remove the fat from the liquids, dump any liquid from the pan into another dish. Then place the juices back in the pan and start cutting the pork roast into medium-sized chunks and scraping any big fat or tendon pieces

Spray the same rub you cooked with over the pulled bits to provide a few extra spices and spray it with the cooking sauces

Combine all coleslaw dressing components and check taste for further changes to the seasoning. Toss the coleslaw (or cabbage mix) with the sauce. Coleslaw may appear thicker to begin with but will change for 1 hour while resting in the fridge

Heat waffle iron for waffles. Drop one slice of cheese onto the waffle iron or scatter grated mozzarella cheese to cover the waffle maker's rim. Place 1/2 of a devilled egg over the cheese, which might melt. Place segmented cheese slice or cover with grated cheese and cover waffle iron. If you like it to be crunchier, let it steam for 3 minutes (until sides crisp) or more. When it cools, it can become crunchier, so check first to see what consistency you want and then change the period accordingly

Place chaffle sandwich together or eat in a bowl if you like to skip the chaffles

1. Use this remaining pulled pork at lunch for the next two days

Nutritional INFO:

1000 kcal Calories | 48g Fat | 70g Carbs | 88g Proteins

Blue Cheese Chaffle Bites

Servings: 2

Cooking Time: 14 Minutes

Ingredients:

- 1 egg, beaten
- ½ cup finely grated Parmesan cheese
- ¼ cup crumbled blue cheese
- 1 tsp erythritol

Directions:

Preheat the waffle iron.

Mix all the ingredients in a bowl.

Open the iron and add half of the mixture. Close and cook until crispy, 7 minutes.

Remove the chaffle onto a plate and make another with the remaining mixture.

Cut each chaffle into wedges and serve afterward.

Nutrition Info:

Per Servings: Calories 19 | Fats 13.91g | Carbs 4.03g

Net Carbs 4.03g | Protein 13.48g

Keto Coffee Cake Chaffle

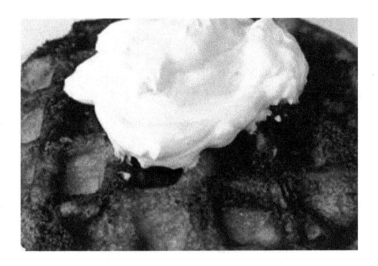

Servings: 4-5

Preparation time: 20-25 minutes

Ingredients
For Chaffle:

- 1 tbsp of butter
- 1 egg
- 1/2 tsp of vanilla
- 2 tbsp of almond flour
- 1 tbsp of coconut flour
- 1/8 tsp of baking powder
- 1 tbsp of Monk fruit For

Crumble:

- 1/2 tsp of cinnamon
- 1 tbsp of melted butter
- 1 tsp of Monk Fruit (or any other sweetener)
- 1 tbsp of chopped pecans

Instructions

Chaffle: In a bowl, melt the butter and mix it with the vanilla and the egg. Then combine in the remainder of the chaffle ingredients

Crumble: in some other bowl having the butter (melted) for crumble, insert and blend the remaining ingredients

Put half the mixture into your griddle or waffle maker
Topping with half of the mixture of crumble

Cook for 5 minutes or till completed

Repeat for all the other components

Just let chaffle cool a bit before the frosting is spread on the chaffle

Nutritional Info:

391 kcal Calories | 35 g Fat | 8 g Carbs | 10 g Proteins

Raspberries Chaffles

Servings:2

Cooking Time: 5 Minutes

Ingredients:

- 1 egg
- 1/2 cup mozzarella cheese, shredded
- 1 tbsp. almond flour
- 1/4 cup raspberry puree
- 1 tbsp. coconut flour for topping

Directions:

Preheat your waffle makerin line with the manufacturer's instructions. Grease your waffle maker with cooking spray.

Mix together egg, almond flour, and raspberry purée. Add cheese and mix until well combined.

Pour batter into the waffle maker. Close the lid.

Cook for about 3-4-minute sutes or until waffles are cooked and not soggy.

Once cooked, remove from the maker. Sprinkle coconut flour on top and enjoy!

Nutrition Info:

Per Servings: Protein: 26% 60 kcal | Fat: 63% 145 kcal | Carbohydrates: 11% 25 kcal

Simple Chaffle Toast

Servings:2

Cooking Time: 5 Minutes

Ingredients:

- 1 large egg
- 1/2 cup shredded cheddar cheese
- FOR TOPPING
- 1 egg
- 3-4 spinach leaves
- ¼ cup boil and shredded chicken

Directions:

Preheat your square waffle maker on medium-high heat.

Mix together egg and cheese in a bowl and make two chaffles in a chaffle maker

Once chaffle are cooked, carefully remove them from the maker. Serve with spinach, boiled chicken, and fried egg.

Serve hot and enjoy!

Nutrition Info:

Per Servings: Protein: 39% 99 kcal | Fat: % 153 kcal

Carbohydrates: 1% 3 kcal

Savory Beef Chaffle

Servings: 2

Cooking Time: 15 Minutes

Ingredients:

- 1 teaspoon olive oil
- 2 cups ground beef
- Garlic salt to taste
- 1 red bell pepper, sliced into strips
- 1 green bell pepper, sliced into strips
- 1 onion, minced
- 1 bay leaf
- 2 garlic chaffles
- Butter

Directions:

Put your pan over medium heat. Add the olive oil and cook ground beef until brown. Season with garlic salt and add bay leaf.

Drain the fat, transfer to a plate and set aside. Discard the bay leaf.

In the same pan, cook the onion and bell peppers for 2 minutes. Put the beef back to the pan.

Heat for 1 minute. Spread butter on top of the chaffle. Add the ground beef and veggies. Roll or fold the chaffle.

Nutrition Info: Calories 220 | Total Fat 17.8g | Saturated Fat 8g

Cholesterol 76mg | Sodium 60mg | Total Carbohydrate 3g | Dietary

Fiber 2g | Total Sugars 5.4g | Protein 27.1g | Potassium 537mg

Chaffles With Almond Flour

Servings:4

Cooking Time: 5 Minutes

Ingredients:

- 2 large eggs
- 1/4 cup almond flour
- 3/4 tsp baking powder
- 1 cup cheddar cheese, shredded
- Cooking spray

Directions:

Switch on your waffle maker and grease with cooking spray.

Beat eggs with almond flour and baking powder in a mixing bowl. Once the eggs and cheese are mixed together, add in cheese and mix again.

Pour 1/cup of the batter in the dash mini waffle maker and close the lid. Cook chaffles for about 2-3 minutes until crispy and cooked

Repeat with the remaining batter Carefully transfer the chafflesto plate. Serve with almonds and enjoy!

Nutrition Info:

Per Servings: Protein: 23% 52 kcal | Fat: 72% 15kcal | Carbohydrates: 5% 11 kcal

Nutter Butter Chaffles

Servings: 2

Cooking Time: 14 Minutes

Ingredients:

- For the chaffles:
- 2 tbsp sugar-free peanut butter powder
- 2 tbsp maple (sugar-free) syrup
- 1 egg, beaten
- ¼ cup finely grated mozzarella cheese
- ¼ tsp baking powder
- ¼ tsp almond butter
- ¼ tsp peanut butter extract
- 1 tbsp softened cream cheese
- For the frosting:
- ½ cup almond flour
- 1 cup peanut butter
- 3 tbsp almond milk
- ½ tsp vanilla extract
- ½ cup maple (sugar-free) syrup

Directions:

Preheat the waffle iron.

Meanwhile, in a medium bowl, mix all the ingredients until smooth. Open the iron and pour in half of the mixture.

Close the iron and cook until crispy, 6 to 7 minutes. Remove the chaffle onto a plate and set aside.

Make a second chaffle with the remaining batter. While the chaffles cool, make the frosting.

Pour the almond flour in a medium saucepan and stir-fry over medium heat until golden.

Transfer the almond flour to a blender and top with the remaining frosting ingredients. Process until smooth.

Spread the frosting on the chaffles and serve afterward.

Nutrition Info:

Calories 239 | Fats 15.48g |Carbs 17.42g | Net Carbs 15.92g | Protein 7.52g

Hot Dog Chaffles

Servings: 2

Cooking Time: 14 Minutes

Ingredients:

- 1 egg, beaten
- 1 cup finely grated cheddar cheese
- 2 hot dog sausages, cooked
- Mustard dressing for topping
- 8 pickle slices

Directions:

Preheat the waffle iron.

In a medium bowl, mix the egg and cheddar cheese.

Open the iron and add half of the mixture. Close and cook until crispy, 7 minutes.

Transfer the chaffle to a plate and make a second chaffle in the same manner.

To serve, top each chaffle with a sausage, swirl the mustard dressing on top, and then divide the pickle slices on top.

Enjoy!

Nutrition Info:

Calories 231 | Fats 18.29g | Carbs 2.8g | Net Carbs 2.6g

Protein 13.39g

Keto Tuna Chaffle Sandwich

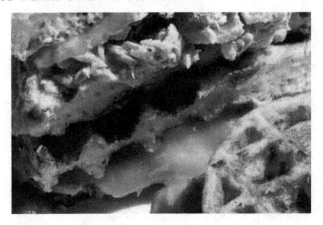

Servings: 1-2

Preparation time: 20 minutes

Ingredients

- 1 egg
- 3/4 cup of almond flour
- 1/2 tsp baking powder
- 1/8 t of salt
- 2 tbsp melted butter
- 1/4 cup mozzarella shredded cheese
- 1/4 cup sour cream

Directions

Mix together the ingredients and place the batter into a mini waffle iron to produce a batch of chaffles

Tuna Sandwich: Take two chaffles and bring together to make a sandwich with your St. Jude tuna salad. Choose your unique flavour of St. Jude tuna: blend with a little bit of olive oil and pepper. Add pepperoncini, tomatoes, red onion, red peppers and all other preferred toppings

Nutritional Info: 1000 kcal Calories | 37 g Fat | 45 g Carbs | Proteins 96 g

Keto Reuben Chaffles

Servings: 4

Cooking Time: 28 Minutes

Ingredients:

- For the chaffles:
- 2 eggs, beaten
- 1 cup finely grated Swiss cheese
- 2 tsp caraway seeds
- 1/8 tsp salt
- ½ tsp baking powder
- For the sauce:
- 2 tbsp sugar-free ketchup
- 3 tbsp mayonnaise
- 1 tbsp dill relish
- 1 tsp hot sauce
- For the filling:
- 6 oz pastrami
- 2 Swiss cheese slices
- ¼ cup pickled radishes

Directions: For the chaffles: Preheat the waffle iron.

In a medium bowl, mix the eggs, Swiss cheese, caraway seeds, salt, and baking powder.

Open the iron and add a quarter of the mixture. Close and cook until crispy, 7 minutes.

Transfer the chaffle to a plate and make 3 more chaffles in the same manner.

For the sauce: In another bowl, mix the ketchup, mayonnaise, dill relish, and hot sauce.

To assemble: Divide on two chaffles; the sauce, the pastrami, Swiss cheese slices, and pickled radishes.

Cover with the other chaffles, divide the sandwich in halves and serve.

Nutrition Info: Calories 316 | Fats 21.78g | Carbs 6.52g | Net Carbs 5.42g | Protein 23.56g

Carrot Chaffle Cake

Servings: 6

Cooking Time: 24 Minutes

Ingredients:

- 1 egg, beaten
- 2 tablespoons melted butter
- ½ cup carrot, shredded
- ¾ cup almond flour
- 1 teaspoon baking powder
- 2 tablespoons heavy whipping cream
- 2 tablespoons sweetener
- 1 tablespoon walnuts, chopped
- 1 teaspoon pumpkin spice
- 2 teaspoons cinnamon

Directions:

Preheat your waffle maker.

In a large bowl, combine all the ingredients. Pour some of the mixture into the waffle maker. Close and cook for minutes.

Repeat steps until all the remaining batter has been used.

Nutrition Info:

Calories 294 | Total Fat 27g | Saturated Fat 12g | Cholesterol 133mg Sodium 144mg | Potassium 421mg | Total Carbohydrate 11.6g Dietary Fiber 4.5g | Protein 6.8g | Total Sugars 1.7g

Egg & Chives Chaffle Sandwich Roll

Servings: 2

Cooking Time: 0 Minute

Ingredients:

- 2 tablespoons mayonnaise
- 1 hard-boiled egg, chopped
- 1 tablespoon chives, chopped
- 2 basic chaffles

Directions:

In a bowl, mix the mayo, egg and chives. Spread the mixture on top of the chaffles. Roll the chaffle.

Nutrition Info:

Calories 258 | Total Fat 12g | Saturated Fat 2.8g | Cholesterol 171mg Sodium 271mg | Potassium 71mg | Total Carbohydrate 7.5g | Dietary Fiber 0.1g | Protein 5.9g | Total Sugars 2.3g

Basic Chaffles Recipe For Sandwiches

Servings:2

Cooking Time: 5 Minutes

Ingredients:

- 1/2 cup mozzarella cheese, shredded
- 1 large egg
- 2 tbsps. almond flour
- 1/2 tsp psyllium husk powder
- 1/4 tsp baking powder

Directions:

Grease your Belgian waffle maker with cooking spray.

Beat the egg with a fork; once the egg is beaten, add almond flour, husk powder, and baking powder.

Add cheese to the egg mixture and mix until combined. Pour batter in the center of Belgian waffle and close the lid. Cook chaffles for about 2-3-minute sutes until well cooked. Carefully transfer the chaffles to plate.

The chaffles are perfect for a sandwich base.

Nutrition Info:

Per Servings: Protein: 29% 60 kcal | Fat: 63% 132 kcal| Carbohydrates: 18 kcal

Okonomiyaki Chaffles

Servings: 4

Cooking Time: 28 Minutes

Ingredients:

- For the chaffles:
- 2 eggs, beaten
- 1 cup finely grated mozzarella cheese
- ½ tsp baking powder
- ¼ cup shredded radishes
- For the sauce:
- 2 tsp coconut aminos
- 2 tbsp sugar-free ketchup
- 1 tbsp sugar-free maple syrup
- 2 tsp Worcestershire sauce
- For the topping:
- 1 tbsp mayonnaise
- 2 tbsp chopped fresh scallions
- 2 tbsp bonito flakes
- 1 tsp dried seaweed powder
- 1 tbsp pickled ginger

Directions:

For the chaffles:

Preheat the waffle iron.

In a medium bowl, mix the eggs, mozzarella cheese, baking powder, and radishes.

Open the iron and add a quarter of the mixture. Close and cook until crispy, 7 minutes.

Transfer the chaffle to a plate and make a 3 more chaffles in the same manner.

For the sauce:

Combine the coconut aminos, ketchup, maple syrup, and Worcestershire sauce in a medium bowl and mix well.

For the topping:

In another mixing bowl, mix the mayonnaise, scallions, bonito flakes, seaweed powder, and ginger

To Servings:

Arrange the chaffles on four different plates and swirl the sauce on top. Spread the topping on the chaffles and serve afterward.

Nutrition Info:

Calories 90 | Fats 3.32g | Carbs 2.97g | Net Carbs 2.17g | Protein 09g

Bacon & Chicken Ranch Chaffle

Servings: 2

Cooking Time: 8 Minutes

Ingredients:

- 1 egg
- ¼ cup chicken cubes, cooked
- 1 slice bacon, cooked and chopped
- ¼ cup cheddar cheese, shredded
- 1 teaspoon ranch dressing powder

Directions:

Preheat your waffle maker.

In a bowl, mix all the ingredients.

Add half of the mixture to your waffle maker. Cover and cook for minutes.

Make the second chaffle using the same steps.

Nutrition Info:

Calories 200Total | Fat 14 g | Saturated Fat g | Cholesterol 129 mg Sodium 463 mg | Potassium 130 mg | Total Carbohydrate 2 g Dietary Fiber 1 g | Protein 16 g | Total Sugars 1 g

Keto Cocoa Chaffles

Servings:2

Cooking Time: 5 Minutes

Ingredients:

- 1 large egg
- 1/2 cup shredded cheddar cheese
- 1 tbsp. cocoa powder
- 2 tbsps. almond flour

Directions:

Preheat your round waffle maker on medium-high heat.

Mix together egg, cheese, almond flour, cocoa powder and vanilla in a small mixing bowl.

Pour chaffles mixture into the center of the waffle iron.

Close the waffle maker and let cook for 3-5 minutesutes or until waffle is golden brown and set.

Carefully remove chaffles from the waffle maker.

Serve hot and enjoy!

Nutrition Info:

Per Servings: Protein: 20% 49 kcal | Fat: % 183 kcal | Carbohydrates: 7% 17 kcal

Keto Chaffle Glazed Donut

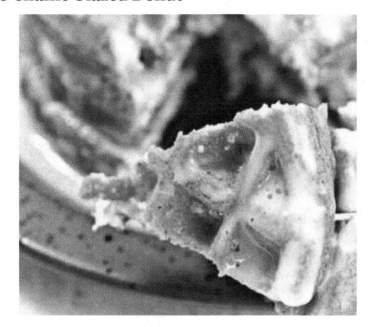

Servings: 2-3

Preparation Time: 10 min

Ingredients

For the chaffles

- ½ cup of shredded mozzarella cheese
- 1 oz. of cream cheese
- 2 tbsp of unflavored protein whey isolate
- 2 tbsp of sugar substitute, swerve confectioners
- ½ tsp of baking powder
- ½ tsp of vanilla extract
- 1 egg

For the topping of glaze:

- 2 tbsp of whipping cream, heavy
- 3-4 tbsp of sugar substitute, swerve confectioners
- ½ tsp of vanilla extract

Directions

Preheat the waffle maker

Mix the cream cheese, and mozzarella cheese in a microwave protected bowl

Heat at the intervals of 30 seconds till the cheeses become melt and mix in completely

Insert 2 tablespoons Swerve sweetener, baking powder and whey protein to the cheese mixture, then knead till it's merged well

Put the dough in a bowl and, till a gentle batter is formed, beat the vanilla and egg

Put one-third of the batter in the waffle maker (mini) and cook for 3 to 5 min until you have attained your required level of doneness

Repeat the fifth step with the batter's left 2/3, with such a total of 3 produced chaffles

Mix together all of the ingredients for glaze topping, & spill over the chaffles prior to serving

Nutritional Info:

75 kcal Calories | 3 g Fat | 2 g Carbs| 5 g Proteins

Barbecue Chaffle

Servings: 2

Cooking Time: 8 Minutes

Ingredients:

- 1 egg, beaten
- ½ cup cheddar cheese, shredded
- ½ teaspoon barbecue sauce
- ¼ teaspoon baking powder

Directions:

Plug in your waffle maker to preheat. Mix all the ingredients in a bowl.

Pour half of the mixture to your waffle maker. Cover and cook for minutes.

Repeat the same steps for the next barbecue chaffle.

Nutrition Info:

Calories 295 | Total Fat 23 g | Saturated Fat 13 g | Cholesterol 223 mg | Sodium 414 mg | Potassium 179 mg | Total Carbohydrate 2 g Dietary Fiber 1 g | Protein 20 g | Total Sugars 1 g

Colby Jack Slices Chaffles

Servings: 1

Cooking Time: 6 Minutes

Ingredients:

- 2 ounces Colby Jack cheese, cut into thin triangle slices
- 1 large organic egg, beaten

Directions:

Preheat a waffle iron and then grease it.

Arrange 1 thin layer of cheese slices in the bottom of preheated waffle iron.

Place the beaten egg on top of the cheese.

Now, arrange another layer of cheese slice on top to cover evenly. Cook for about 6 minutes or until golden brown.

Serve warm.

Nutrition Info:

Per Servings: Calories: 292 | Net Carb: 2.4g | Fat: 23g Saturated

Fat: 13.6g | Carbohydrates: 2.4g | Dietary Fiber: 0g | Sugar: 0.4g

Protein: 18.3g

Chicken And Chaffle Nachos

Servings: 4

Cooking Time: 33 Minutes

Ingredients:

- For the chaffles:
- 2 eggs, beaten
- 1 cup finely grated Mexican cheese blend
- For the chicken-cheese topping:
- 2 tbsp butter
- 1 tbsp almond flour
- ¼ cup unsweetened almond milk
- 1 cup finely grated cheddar cheese + more to garnish
- 3 bacon slices, cooked and chopped
- 2 cups cooked and diced chicken breasts
- 2 tbsp hot sauce
- 2 tbsp chopped fresh scallions

Directions:
For the chaffles:

Preheat the waffle iron.

In a medium bowl, mix the eggs and Mexican cheese blend.

Open the iron and add a quarter of the mixture. Close and cook until crispy, 7 minutes.

Transfer the chaffle to a plate and make 3 more chaffles in the same manner.

Place the chaffles on serving plates and set aside for serving.

For the chicken-cheese topping:

Melt the butter in a large skillet and mix in the almond flour until brown, 1 minute.

Pour the almond milk and whisk until well combined. Simmer until thickened, 2 minutes.

Stir in the cheese to melt, 2 minutes and then mix in the bacon, chicken, and hot sauce.

Spoon the mixture onto the chaffles and top with some more cheddar cheese.

Garnish with the scallions and serve immediately.

Nutrition Info:

Calories 524 | Fats 37.51g | Carbs 3.55g | Net Carbs 3.25g | Protein 41.86g

Ham, Cheese & Tomato Chaffle Sandwich

Servings: 2

Cooking Time: 10 Minutes

Ingredients:

- 1 teaspoon olive oil
- 2 slices ham
- 4 basic chaffles
- 1 tablespoon mayonnaise
- 2 slices Provolone cheese
- 1 tomato, sliced

Directions:

Add the olive oil to a pan over medium heat. Cook the ham for 1 minute per side.

Spread the chaffles with mayonnaise. Top with the ham, cheese and tomatoes.

Top with another chaffle to make a sandwich.

Nutrition Info:

Calories 198 | Total Fat 14.7g | Saturated Fat 3g | Cholesterol 37mg Sodium 664mg | Total Carbohydrate 4.6g | Dietary Fiber 0.7g | Total Sugars 1.5g | Protein 12.2g | Potassium 193mg

Cereal Chaffle Cake

Servings: 2

Cooking Time: 8 Minutes

Ingredients:

- 1 egg
- 2 tablespoons almond flour
- ½ teaspoon coconut flour
- 1 tablespoon melted butter
- 1 tablespoon cream cheese
- 1 tablespoon plain cereal, crushed
- ¼ teaspoon vanilla extract
- ¼ teaspoon baking powder
- 1 tablespoon sweetener
- 1/8 teaspoon xanthan gum

Directions:

Plug in your waffle maker to preheat. Add all the ingredients in a large bowl. Mix until well blended.

Let the batter rest for 2 minutes before cooking. Pour half of the mixture into the waffle maker. Seal and cook for 4 minutes.

Make the next chaffle using the same steps.

Nutrition Info:

Calories154 | Total Fat 21.2g | Saturated Fat 10 g | Cholesterol 113.3mg | Sodium 96.9mg | Potassium 453 mg | Total Carbohydrate 5.9g | Dietary Fiber 1.7g | Protein 4.6g | Total Sugars 2.7g

Sweet Chaffles Recipes

Lemon Curd Chaffles Servings: 1

Cooking Time: 5 Minutes

Ingredients:

- 3 large eggs
- 4 oz cream cheese, softened
- 1 Tbsp low carb sweetener
- 1 tsp vanilla extract
- ¾ cup mozzarella cheese, shredded
- 3 Tbsp coconut flour
- 1 tsp baking powder
- ⅓ tsp salt
- For the lemon curd:
- ½-1 cup water
- 5 egg yolks
- ½ cup lemon juice
- ½ cup powdered sweetener
- 2 Tbsp fresh lemon zest
- 1 tsp vanilla extract
- Pinch of salt
- 8 Tbsp cold butter, cubed

Directions:

Pour water into a saucepan and heat over medium until it reaches a soft boil. Start with ½ cup and add more if needed.

Whisk yolks, lemon juice, lemon zest, powdered sweetener, vanilla, and salt in a medium heat-proof bowl. Leave to set for 5-6 minutes.

Place bowl onto saucepan and heat. The bowl shouldn't be touching water.

Whisk mixture for 8-10 minutes, or until it begins to thicken. Add butter cubes and whisk for 7 minutes, until it thickens. When it lightly coats the back of a spoon, remove from heat. Refrigerate until cool, allowing it to continue thickening.

Turn on waffle maker to heat and oil it with cooking spray.

Add baking powder, coconut flour, and salt in a small bowl. Mix well and set aside.

Add eggs, cream cheese, sweetener, and vanilla in a separate bowl. Using a hand beater, beat until frothy.

Add mozzarella to egg mixture and beat again. Add dry ingredients and mix until well-combined.

Add batter to waffle maker and cook for 3-4 minutes. Transfer to a plate and top with lemon curd before serving.

Nutrition Info:

Carbs: 6 g | Fat: 24 g | Protein: Calories 302

Protein Mozzarella Chaffles

Servings: 4

Cooking Time: 20 Minutes

Ingredients:

- ½ scoop unsweetened protein powder
- 2 large organic eggs
- ½ cup Mozzarella cheese, shredded
- 1 tablespoon Erythritol
- ¼ teaspoon organic vanilla extract

Directions:

Preheat a mini waffle iron and then grease it.

In a medium bowl, place all ingredients and with a fork, mix until well combined.

Place ¼ of the mixture into preheated waffle iron and cook for about 4-5 minutes or until golden brown.

Repeat with the remaining mixture.
Serve warm.

Nutrition Info:

Per Servings: Calories: Net Carb 0.4g | Fat: 3.3g Saturated | Fat: 1.2g | Carbohydrates: 0.4g | Dietary Fiber: 0g | Sugar: 0.2g | Protein: 7.3g

Peanut Butter Chaffles

Servings: 2

Cooking Time: 8 Minutes

Ingredients:

- 1 organic egg, beaten
- ½ cup Mozzarella cheese, shredded
- 3 tablespoons granulated Erythritol
- 2 tablespoons peanut butter

Directions:

Preheat a mini waffle iron and then grease it.

In a medium bowl, place all ingredients and with a fork, mix until well combined.

Place half of the mixture into preheated waffle iron and cook for about 4 minutes or until golden brown.

Repeat with the remaining mixture. Serve warm.

Nutrition Info:

Per Servings: Calories: 145 | Net Carb: 2. | Fat: 11.5g | Saturated Fat: 3.1g | Carbohydrates: 3.6g | Dietary Fiber: 1g Sugar: 1.7g | Protein: 8.8g

Cinnamon Pecan Chaffles

Servings: 1

Cooking Time: 40 Minutes

Ingredients:

- 1 Tbsp butter
- 1 egg
- ½ tsp vanilla
- 2 Tbsp almond flour
- 1 Tbsp coconut flour
- ⅛ tsp baking powder
- 1 Tbsp monk fruit
- For the crumble:
- ½ tsp cinnamon
- 1 Tbsp melted butter
- 1 tsp monk fruit
- 1 Tbsp chopped pecans

Directions:

Turn on waffle maker to heat and oil it with cooking spray.
Melt butter in a bowl, then mix in the egg and vanilla.

Mix in remaining chaffle ingredients.

Combine crumble ingredients in a separate bowl.

Pour half of the chaffle mix into waffle maker. Top with half of
crumble mixture.

Cook for 5 minutes, or until done. Repeat
with the other half of the batter.

Nutrition Info:

Carbs: g | Fat: 35 g | Protein: 10 g | Calories: 391

Simple Mozzarella Chaffles

Servings: 2

Cooking Time: 8 Minutes

Ingredients:

- ½ cup mozzarella cheese, shredded
- 1 large organic egg
- 2 tablespoons blanched almond flour
- ¼ teaspoon organic baking powder
- 2–3 drops liquid stevia

Directions:

Preheat a mini waffle iron and then grease it.

In a medium bowl, put all ingredients and with a fork, mix until well combined. Place half of the mixture into preheated waffle iron and cook for about 3–4 minutes.

Repeat with the remaining mixture. Serve warm.

Nutrition Info:

Calories 98 | Net Carbs 1.4 g | Total Fat 7.1 g | Saturated Fat 1.8 g | Cholesterol 97 mg | Sodium 81 mg | Total Carbs 2.2 g | Fiber 0.8 g | Sugar 0.2 g | Protein 6.7 g

Oreo Keto Chaffles

Servings: 2

Cooking Time: 5 Minutes

Ingredients:

- 1 egg
- 1½ Tbsp unsweetened cocoa
- 2 Tbsp lakanto monk fruit, or choice of sweetener
- 1 Tbsp heavy cream
- 1 tsp coconut flour
- ½ tsp baking powder
- ½ tsp vanilla
- For the cheese cream:
- 1 Tbsp lakanto powdered sweetener
- 2 Tbsp softened cream cheese
- ¼ tsp vanilla

Directions:

Turn on waffle maker to heat and oil it with cooking spray. Combine all chaffle ingredients in a small bowl.

Pour one half of the chaffle mixture into waffle maker.

Cook for 5 minutes.

Remove and repeat with the second half if the mixture. Let chaffles sit for 2-3 to crisp up.

Combine all cream ingredients and spread on chaffle when they have cooled to room temperature.

Nutrition Info:

Carbs: 3 g | Fat: 4 g | Protein: 7 g |

Chocolate Chips Peanut Butter Chaffles

Servings: 2

Cooking Time: 8 Minutes

Ingredients:

- 1 organic egg, beaten
- ¼ cup Mozzarella cheese, shredded
- 2 tablespoons creamy peanut butter
- 1 tablespoon almond flour
- 1 tablespoon granulated Erythritol
- 1 teaspoon organic vanilla extract
- 1 tablespoon 70% dark chocolate chips

Directions:

Preheat a mini waffle iron and then grease it.

In a bowl, place all ingredients except chocolate chips and beat until well combined.

Gently, fold in the chocolate chips.

Place half of the mixture into preheated waffle iron and cook for about minutes or until golden brown.

Repeat with the remaining mixture.
Serve warm.

Nutrition Info:

Per Servings: Calories: 214 | Net Carb: 4.1g | Fat: 16.8g Saturated Fat: 5.4g | Carbohydrates: 6.4g | Dietary Fiber: 2.3g | Sugar: 2.1g | Protein: 8.8g

Mayonnaise Chaffles

Servings: 2

Cooking Time: 10 Minutes

Ingredients:

- 1 large organic egg, beaten1 tablespoon mayonnaise
- 2 tablespoons almond flour
- 1/8 teaspoon organic baking powder
- 1 teaspoon water2–4 drops liquid stevia

Directions:

Preheat a mini waffle iron and then grease it.

In a medium bowl, put all ingredients and with a fork, mix until well combined.

Place half of the mixture into preheated waffle iron and cook for about 4–5 minutes.

Repeat with the remaining mixture.

Serve warm.

Nutrition Info:

Calories 110 | Net Carbs 2.6 g | Total Fat 8.7 g | Saturated Fat 1.4 g | Cholesterol 9mg | Sodium 88 g | Total Carbs 3.4 g | Fiber 0.8 g | Sugar 0.9 g | Protein 3.2 g

Blackberry Chaffles

Servings: 2

Cooking Time: 8 Minutes

Ingredients:

- 1 organic egg, beaten
- 1/3 cup Mozzarella cheese, shredded
- 1 teaspoon cream cheese, softened
- 1 teaspoon coconut flour
- ¼ teaspoon organic baking powder
- ¾ teaspoon powdered Erythritol
- ¼ teaspoon ground cinnamon
- ¼ teaspoon organic vanilla extract
- Pinch of salt
- 1 tablespoon fresh blackberries

Directions:

Preheat a mini waffle iron and then grease it.

In a bowl, place all ingredients except for blackberries and beat until well combined.

Fold in the blackberries.

Place half of the mixture into preheated waffle iron and cook for about minutes or until golden brown.

Repeat with the remaining mixture. Serve warm.

Nutrition Info:

Per Servings: Calories: 121 | Net Carb: 2. | Fat: 7.5g Saturated | Fat: 3.3g | Carbohydrates: 4.5g | Dietary Fiber: 1.8g | Sugar: 0.9g Protein: 8.9g

Chocolate Chips Chaffles

Servings: 2

Cooking Time: 8 Minutes

Ingredients:

- 1 large organic egg
- 1 teaspoon coconut flour
- 1 teaspoon Erythritol
- ½ teaspoon organic vanilla extract
- ½ cup Mozzarella cheese, shredded finely
- 2 tablespoons 70% dark chocolate chips

Directions:

Preheat a mini waffle iron and then grease it.

In a bowl, place the egg, coconut flour, sweetener and vanilla extract and beat until well combined.

Add the cheese and stir to combine.

Place half of the mixture into preheated waffle iron and top with half of the chocolate chips.

Place a little egg mixture over each chocolate chip. Cook for about 3-4 minutes or until golden brown. Repeat with the remaining mixture and chocolate chips. Serve warm.

Nutrition Info:

Per Servings: Calories: 164 | Net Carb: 2. | Fat: 11.9g | Saturated Fat: 6.6g | Carbohydrates: 5.4g | Dietary Fiber: 2.5g | Sugar: 0.3g | Protein: 7.3g

Raspberry Chaffles

Servings: 2

Cooking Time: 5 Minutes

Ingredients:

- 4 Tbsp almond flour
- 4 large eggs
- 2⅓ cup shredded mozzarella cheese
- 1 tsp vanilla extract
- 1 Tbsp erythritol sweetener
- 1½ tsp baking powder
- ½ cup raspberries

Directions:

Turn on waffle maker to heat and oil it with cooking spray. Mix almond flour, sweetener, and baking powder in a bowl.

Add cheese, eggs, and vanilla extract, and mix until well-combined. Add 1 portion of batter to waffle maker and spread it evenly. Close and cook for 3-minutes, or until golden.

Repeat until remaining batter is used.
Serve with raspberries.

Nutrition Info:

Carbs: 5 g | Fat: 11 g | Protein: 24 g | Calories: 300

Mozzarella & Butter Chaffles

Servings: 2

Cooking Time: 8 Minutes

Ingredients:

- 1 large organic egg, beaten
- ¾ cup Mozzarella cheese, shredded
- ½ tablespoon unsalted butter, melted
- 2 tablespoons blanched almond flour
- 2 tablespoons Erythritol
- ½ teaspoon ground cinnamon
- ½ teaspoon Psyllium husk powder
- ¼ teaspoon organic baking powder
- ½ teaspoon organic vanilla extract

Directions:

Preheat a waffle iron and then grease it.

In a medium bowl, place all ingredients and with a fork, mix until well combined.

Place half of the mixture into preheated waffle iron and cook for about 5 minutes or until golden brown.

Repeat with the remaining mixture.
Serve warm.

Nutrition Info:

Per Servings: Calories: 140 | Net Carb: 1.9g | Fat: 10. | Saturated Fat: 4g | Carbohydrates: 3g | Dietary Fiber: 1.1g | Sugar: 0.3g Protein: 7.8g

Layered Chaffles

Servings: 2

Cooking Time: 10 Minutes

Ingredients:

- 1 organic egg, beaten and divided
- ½ cup cheddar cheese, shredded and divided
- Pinch of salt

Directions:

Preheat a mini waffle iron and then grease it.

Place about 1/8 cup of cheese in the bottom of the waffle iron and top with half of the beaten egg.

Now, place 1/8 cup of cheese on top and cook for about 4–5 minutes. Repeat with the remaining cheese and egg.

Serve warm.

Nutrition Info:

Calories 145 | Net Carbs 0.5 g | Total Fat 11.g | Saturated Fat 6.6 g | Cholesterol 112 mg | Sodium 284 g | Total Carbs 0.5 g | Fiber 0 g | Sugar 0.3 g | Protein 9.8 g

Basic Keto Chaffles

Servings: 2

Cooking Time: 5 Minutes

Ingredients:

*   1 egg
*   ½ cup shredded Cheddar cheese

Directions:

Turn on waffle maker to heat and oil it with cooking spray. Whisk egg in a bowl until well beaten.

Add cheese to the egg and stir well to combine.

Pour ½ batter into the waffle maker and close the top. Cook for 3-5 min- utes.

Transfer chaffle to a plate and set aside for 2-3 minutes to crisp up. Repeat for remaining batter.

Nutrition Info:

Carbs: 1 g | Fat: 12 g |Protein: 9 g | Calories: 150

Lemon Chaffles

Servings: 2

Cooking Time: 10 Minutes

Ingredients:

- 1 organic egg, beaten
- 1-ounce cream cheese, softened
- 2 tablespoons almond flour
- 1 tablespoon fresh lemon juice
- 2 teaspoons Erythritol
- ½ teaspoon fresh lemon zest, grated
- ¼ teaspoon organic baking powder
- Pinch of salt
- ½ teaspoon powdered Erythritol

Directions:

Preheat a mini waffle iron and then grease it.

In a bowl, place all ingredients except the powdered Erythritol and beat until well combined.

Place half of the mixture into preheated waffle iron and cook for about 5 minutes or until golden brown.

Repeat with the remaining mixture.

Serve warm with the sprinkling of powdered Erythritol.

Nutrition Info:

Per Servings: Calories: 129 | Net Carb: 1.2g |Fat: 10.9g | Saturated Fat: 4.1g | Carbohydrates: 2.4g | Dietary Fiber: 0.8g | Sugar: 0 Protein: 3.9g

Chocolate Chip Chaffles

Servings: 1

Cooking Time: 6 Minutes

Ingredients:

- 1 egg
- 1 tsp coconut flour
- 1 tsp sweetener
- ½ tsp vanilla extract
- ¼ cup heavy whipping cream, for serving
- ½ cup almond milk ricotta, finely shredded
- 2 tbsp sugar-free chocolate chips

Directions:

Preheat your mini waffle iron.

Mix the egg, coconut flour, vanilla, and sweetener. Whisk together with a fork.

Stir in the almond milk ricotta.

Pour half of the batter into the waffle iron and dot with a pinch of chocolate chips.

Close the waffle iron and cook for minutes. Repeat with remaining batter.

Serve hot with the whipped cream.

Nutrition Info:

Calories Per Servings:

304 Kcal |Fats: 16 g | Carbs: 7g | Protein: 3 g

Banana Nut Chaffle

Servings: 1

Cooking Time: 10 Minutes

Ingredients:

- 1 egg
- 1 Tbsp cream cheese, softened and room temp
- 1 Tbsp sugar-free cheesecake pudding
- ½ cup mozzarella cheese
- 1 Tbsp monk fruit confectioners' sweetener
- ¼ tsp vanilla extract
- ¼ tsp banana extract
- toppings of choice

Directions:

Turn on waffle maker to heat and oil it with cooking spray. Beat egg in a small bowl.

Add remaining ingredients and mix until well incorporated.

Add one half of the batter to waffle maker and cook for minutes, until golden brown.

Remove chaffle and add the other half of the batter. Top with your optional toppings and serve warm!

Nutrition Info:

Carbs: 2 g | Protein: 8 g | Calories: 119

Pumpkin Cream Cheese Chaffles

Servings: 2

Cooking Time: 10 Minutes

Ingredients:

- 1 organic egg, beaten
- ½ cup Mozzarella cheese, shredded
- 1½ tablespoon sugar-free pumpkin puree
- 2 teaspoons heavy cream
- 1 teaspoon cream cheese, softened
- 1 tablespoon almond flour
- 1 tablespoon Erythritol
- ½ teaspoon pumpkin pie spice
- ½ teaspoon organic baking powder
- 1 teaspoon organic vanilla extract

Directions:

Preheat a mini waffle iron and then grease it.

In a medium bowl, place all ingredients and with a fork, mix until well combined.

Place half of the mixture into preheated waffle iron and cook for about 5 minutes or until golden brown.

Repeat with the remaining mixture.
Serve warm.

Nutrition Info:

Per Servings: Calories: 110 | Net Carb: 2.5g | Fat: 4.3g | Saturated Fat: 1g | Carbohydrates: 3.3g | Dietary Fiber: 0.8g | Sugar: 1g Protein: 5.2g

Whipping Cream Pumpkin Chaffles

Servings: 4

Cooking Time: 12 Minutes

Ingredients:

- 2 organic eggs
- 2 tablespoons homemade pumpkin puree
- 2 tablespoons heavy whipping cream
- 1 tablespoon coconut flour
- 1 tablespoon Erythritol
- 1 teaspoon pumpkin pie spice
- ½ teaspoon organic baking powder
- ½ teaspoon organic vanilla extract
- Pinch of salt
- ½ cup Mozzarella cheese, shredded

Directions:

Preheat a mini waffle iron and then grease it.

In a bowl, place all the ingredients except Mozzarella cheese and beat until well combined.

Add the Mozzarella cheese and stir to combine.

Place half of the mixture into preheated waffle iron and cook for about 6 minutes or until golden brown.

Repeat with the remaining mixture. Serve warm.

Nutrition Info:

Per Servings: Calories: 81 | Net Carb: 2.1g | Fat: 5.9g | Saturated Fat: 3g | Carbohydrates: 3.1g | Dietary Fiber: 1g Sugar: 0.5g | Protein: 4.3g

Chocolate Chaffles

Servings: 2

Cooking Time: 10 Minutes

Ingredients:

- ¾ cup shredded mozzarella
- 1 large egg
- 2 Tbsp almond flour
- 2 Tbsp allulose
- ½ Tbsp melted butter
- 1½ Tbsp cocoa powder
- ½ tsp vanilla extract
- ½ tsp psyllium husk powder
- ¼ tsp baking powder

Directions:

Turn on waffle maker to heat and oil it with cooking spray.
Mix all ingredients in a small bowl.

Pour ¼ cup batter into a 4-inch waffle maker.
Cook for 2-3 minutes, or until crispy.

Transfer chaffle to a plate and set aside.
Repeat with remaining batter.

Nutrition Info:

Carbs: 6 g | Fat: 24 g | Protein: 15 g | Calories: 296

Chocolate Chips Lemon Chaffles

Servings: 4

Cooking Time: 8 Minutes

Ingredients:

- 2 organic eggs
- ½ cup Mozzarella cheese, shredded
- ¾ teaspoon organic lemon extract
- ½ teaspoon organic vanilla extract
- 2 teaspoons Erythritol
- ½ teaspoon psyllium husk powder
- Pinch of salt
- 1 tablespoon 70% dark chocolate chips
- ¼ teaspoon lemon zest, grated finely

Directions:

Preheat a mini waffle iron and then grease it.

In a bowl, place all ingredients except chocolate chips and lemon zest and beat until well combined.

Gently, fold in the chocolate chips and lemon zest.

Place ¼ of the mixture into preheated waffle iron and cook for about minutes or until golden brown.

Repeat with the remaining mixture.

Serve warm.

Nutrition Info:

Per Servings: Calories: Net Carb: 1g | Fat: 4.8g Saturated Fat: 2.3g | Carbohydrates: 1.5g | Dietary Fiber: 0.5g | Sugar: 0.3g |Protein: 4.3g

Coconut & Walnut Chaffles

Servings: 8

Cooking Time: 24 Minutes

Ingredients:

- 4 organic eggs, beaten
- 4 ounces cream cheese, softened
- 1 tablespoon butter, melted
- 4 tablespoons coconut flour
- 1 tablespoon almond flour
- 2 tablespoons Erythritol
- 1½ teaspoons organic baking powder
- 1 teaspoon organic vanilla extract
- ½ teaspoon ground cinnamon
- 1 tablespoon unsweetened coconut, shredded
- 1 tablespoon walnuts, chopped

Directions:

Preheat a mini waffle iron and then grease it.

In a blender, place all ingredients and pulse until creamy and smooth. Divide the mixture into 8 portions.

Place 1 portion of the mixture into preheated waffle iron and cook for about 2-3 minutes or until golden brown.

Repeat with the remaining mixture.
Serve warm.

Nutrition Info:

Per Servings: Calories: 125 | Net Carb: 2.2g | Fat: 10.2g | Saturated Fat: 5.2g | Carbohydrates: 4g | Dietary Fiber: 1.8g Sugar: 0.4g | Protein: 4.6g

Cream Mini-chaffles

Servings: 2

Cooking Time: 10 Minutes

Ingredients:

- 2 tsp coconut flour
- 4 tsp swerve/monk fruit
- ¼ tsp baking powder
- 1 egg
- 1 oz cream cheese
- ½ tsp vanilla extract

Directions:

Turn on waffle maker to heat and oil it with cooking spray.

Mix swerve/monk fruit, coconut flour, and baking powder in a small mixing bowl.

Add cream cheese, egg, vanilla extract, and whisk until well-combined. Add batter into waffle maker and cook for 3-minutes, until golden brown. Serve with your favourite toppings.

Nutrition Info:

Carbs: 4 g | Protein: 2 g | Calories: 73

Chocolaty Chips Pumpkin Chaffles

Servings: 3

Cooking Time: 12 Minutes

Ingredients:

- 1 organic egg
- 4 teaspoons homemade pumpkin puree
- ½ cup Mozzarella cheese, shredded
- 1 tablespoon almond flour
- 2 tablespoons granulated Erythritol
- ¼ teaspoon pumpkin pie spice
- 4 teaspoons 70% dark chocolate chips

Directions:

In a bowl, place the egg and pumpkin puree and mix well.

Add the remaining ingredients except for chocolate chips and mix until well combined.

Gently, fold in the chocolate chips and lemon zest.

Place 1/3 of the mixture into preheated waffle iron and cook for about minutes or until golden brown.

Repeat with the remaining mixture. Serve warm.

Nutrition Info:

Per Servings: Calories: 9et Carb: 1.9g | Fat: 7.1g | Saturated Fat: 3.3g | Carbohydrates: 1.4g | Dietary Fiber: 2.6g | Sugar: 0.4g | Protein: 4.2g

Vanilla Chaffle

Servings: 2

Cooking Time: 8 Minutes

Ingredients:

- 2 tbsp butter, softened
- 2 oz cream cheese, softened
- 2 eggs
- ¼ cup almond flour
- 2 tbsp coconut flour
- 1 tsp baking powder
- 1 tsp vanilla extract
- ¼ cup confectioners
- Pinch of pink salt

Directions:

Preheat the waffle maker and spray with non-stick cooking spray. Melt the butter and set aside for a minute to cool.

Add the eggs into the melted butter and whisk until creamy. Pour in the sweetener, vanilla, extract, and salt. Blend properly.

Next add the coconut flour, almond flour, and baking powder. Mix well. Pour into the waffle maker and cook for 4 minutes.

Repeat the process with the remaining batter.
Remove and set aside to cool.

Enjoy.

Nutrition Info:

Calories Per Servings: 202 Kcal | Fats: 27 g |Carbs: 9 g | Protein: 23 g

Pumpkin Pecan Chaffles

Servings: 2

Cooking Time: 10 Minutes

Ingredients:

- 1 egg
- ½ cup mozzarella cheese grated
- 1 Tbsp pumpkin puree
- ½ tsp pumpkin spice
- 1 tsp erythritol low carb sweetener
- 2 Tbsp almond flour
- 2 Tbsp pecans, toasted chopped
- 1 cup heavy whipped cream
- ¼ cup low carb caramel sauce

Directions:

Turn on waffle maker to heat and oil it with cooking spray. In a bowl, beat egg.

Mix in mozzarella, pumpkin, flour, pumpkin spice, and erythritol. Stir in pecan pieces.

Spoon one half of the batter into waffle maker and spread evenly. Close and cook for 5 minutes.

Remove cooked waffles to a plate. Repeat with remaining batter.

Serve with pecans, whipped cream, and low carb caramel sauce.

Nutrition Info:

Carbs: 4 g | Fat: 17 g | Protein: 11 g | Calories: 210

Walnut Pumpkin Chaffles

Servings: 2

Cooking Time: 10 Minutes

- 1 organic egg, beaten
- ½ cup Mozzarella cheese, shredded
- 2 tablespoons almond flour
- 1 tablespoon sugar-free pumpkin puree
- 1 teaspoon Erythritol
- ¼ teaspoon ground cinnamon
- 2 tablespoons walnuts, toasted and chopped

Directions:

Preheat a mini waffle iron and then grease it.

In a bowl, place all ingredients except walnuts and beat until well com- bined.

Fold in the walnuts.

Place half of the mixture into preheated waffle iron and cook for about 5 minutes or until golden brown.

Repeat with the remaining mixture.
Serve warm.

Nutrition Info:

Per Servings: Calories: 148 | Net Carb: 1.6g | Fat: 11.8g | Saturated Fat: 2g | Carbohydrates: 3.3g | Dietary Fiber: 1. | Sugar: 0.8g Protein: 6.7g

Chaffle Glazed With Raspberry

Servings: 1

Cooking Time: 5 Minutes

Ingredients:

- Donut Chaffle Ingredients:
- 1 egg
- ¼ cup mozzarella cheese, shredded
- 2 tsp cream cheese, softened
- 1 tsp sweetener
- 1tsp almond flour
- ½ tsp baking powder
- 20 drops glazed donut flavoring
- Raspberry Jelly Filling:
- ¼ cup raspberries
- 1 tsp chia seeds
- 1 tsp confectioners' sweetener
- Donut Glaze:
- 1 tsp powdered sweetener
- Heavy whipping cream

Directions:

1. Spray your waffle maker with cooking oil and add the butter mixture into the waffle maker.
2. Cook for 3 minutes and set aside.
3. Raspberry Jelly Filling:
4. Mix all the
5. Place in a pot and heat on medium.
6. Gently mash the raspberries and set aside to cool.
7. Donut Glaze:
8. Stir together the
9. Assembling:

Lay your chaffles on a plate and add the fillings mixture between the layers.

Drizzle the glaze on top and enjoy.

Nutrition Info:

Calories Per Servings: 188 Kcal | Fats: 23 g | Carbs: 12 g
Protein: 17 g

Chocolate Peanut Butter Chaffle

Servings: 2

Cooking Time: 10 Minutes

Ingredients:

- ½ cup shredded mozzarella cheese
- 1 Tbsp cocoa powder
- 2 Tbsp powdered sweetener
- 2 Tbsp peanut butter
- ½ tsp vanilla
- 1 egg
- 2 Tbsp crushed peanuts
- 2 Tbsp whipped cream
- ¼ cup sugar-free chocolate syrup

Directions:

Combine mozzarella, egg, vanilla, peanut butter, cocoa powder, and sweetener in a bowl.

Add in peanuts and mix well.

Turn on waffle maker and oil it with cooking spray.

Pour one half of the batter into waffle maker and cook for minutes, then transfer to a plate.

Top with whipped cream, peanuts, and sugar-free chocolate syrup.

Nutrition Info:

Fat: 17 g | Protein: 15 g | Calories: 236

Cream Cake Chaffle

Servings: 4

Cooking Time: 12 Minutes

Ingredients:

- Chaffle
- 4 oz cream cheese, softened
- 4 eggs
- 4 tbsp coconut flour
- 1 tbsp almond flour
- 1 ½ tsp baking powder
- 1 tbsp butter, softened
- 1 tsp vanilla extract
- ½ tsp cinnamon
- 1 tbsp sweetener
- 1 tbsp shredded coconut, colored and unsweetened
- 1 tbsp walnuts, chopped
- Italian Cream Frosting
- 2 oz cream cheese, softened
- 2 tbsp butter, room temperature
- 2 tbsp sweetener
- ½ tsp vanilla

Directions:

Preheat your waffle maker and add ¼ of the
Cook for 3 minutes and repeat the process until you have 4 chaffles.
Remove and set aside.
In the meantime, start making your frosting by mixing all the
Stir until you have a smooth and creamy mixture.
Cool, frost the cake and enjoy.

Nutrition Info:

Calories Per Servings: 127 Kcal | Fats: 10 g | Carbs: 5.5 g |
Protein: 7 g

Blueberry Cinnamon Chaffles

Servings: 3

Cooking Time: 10 Minutes

Ingredients:

- 1 cup shredded mozzarella cheese
- 3 Tbsp almond flour
- 2 eggs
- 2 tsp Swerve or granulated sweetener of choice
- 1 tsp cinnamon
- ½ tsp baking powder
- ½ cup fresh blueberries
- ½ tsp of powdered Swerve

Directions:

Turn on waffle maker to heat and oil it with cooking spray.

Mix eggs, flour, mozzarella, cinnamon, vanilla extract, sweetener, and baking powder in a bowl until well combined.

Add in blueberries.

Pour ¼ batter into each waffle mold. Close and cook for 8 minutes.

If it's crispy and the waffle maker opens without pulling the chaffles apart, the chaffle is ready. If not, close and cook for 1-2 minutes more. Serve with favorite topping and more blueberries.

Nutrition Info:

Carbs: 9 g | Fat: 12 g | Protein: 13 g | Calories: 193

Cream Cheese Chaffles

Servings: 2

Cooking Time: 8 Minutes

Ingredients:

- 2 teaspoons coconut flour
- 3 teaspoons Erythritol
- ¼ teaspoon organic baking powder
- 1 organic egg, beaten
- 1-ounce cream cheese, softened
- ½ teaspoon organic vanilla extract

Directions:

Preheat a mini waffle iron and then grease it.

In a bowl, place flour, Erythritol and baking powder and mix well.

Add the egg, cream cheese and vanilla extract and beat until well combined.

Place half of the mixture into preheated waffle iron and cook for about 3-minutes or until golden brown.

Repeat with the remaining mixture.
Serve warm.

Nutrition Info:

Per Servings: Calories: 95 | Net Carb: 1.6g | Fat: 4g | Saturated Fat: 4g | Carbohydrates: 2.6g | Dietary Fiber: 1g | Sugar: 0.3g | Protein: 4.2g

Strawberry Shortcake Chaffles

Servings: 1

Cooking Time: 25 Minutes

Ingredients:

- For the batter:
- 1 egg
- ¼ cup mozzarella cheese
- 1 Tbsp cream cheese
- ¼ tsp baking powder
- 2 strawberries, sliced
- 1 tsp strawberry extract
- For the glaze:
- 1 Tbsp cream cheese
- ¼ tsp strawberry extract
- 1 Tbsp monk fruit confectioners blend
- For the whipped cream:
- 1 cup heavy whipping cream
- 1 tsp vanilla
- 1 Tbsp monk fruit

Directions:

Turn on waffle maker to heat and oil it with cooking spray.
Beat egg in a small bowl.

Add remaining batter components.
Divide the mixture in half.

Cook one half of the batter in a waffle maker for 4 minutes, or until golden brown.

Repeat with remaining batter

Mix all glaze ingredients and spread over each warm chaffle.

Mix all whipped cream ingredients and whip until it starts to form peaks. Top each waffle with whipped cream and strawberries.

Nutrition Info:

Carbs: 5 g | Fat: 14 g | Protein: 12 g | Calories: 218

Chocolate Whipping Cream Chaffles

Servings: 2

Cooking Time: 8 Minutes

Ingredients:

- 1 tablespoon almond flour
- 2 tablespoons cacao powder
- 2 tablespoons granulated Erythritol
- ¼ teaspoon organic baking powder
- 1 organic egg
- 1 tablespoon heavy whipping cream
- ¼ teaspoon organic vanilla extract
- 1/8 teaspoon organic almond extract

Directions:

Preheat a mini waffle iron and then grease it.

In a bowl, place all ingredients and beat until well combined.

Place half of the mixture into preheated waffle iron and cook for about 4 minutes or until golden brown.

Repeat with the remaining mixture. Serve warm.

Nutrition Info:

Per Servings: Calories: 94 | Net Carb: 2g | Fat: 7.9g | Saturated Fat: 3.2g | Carbohydrates: 3.9g | Dietary Fiber: 1.9g | Sugar: 0.4g | Protein: 3.9g

Cream Cheese & Butter Chaffles

Servings: 4

Cooking Time: 16 Minutes

Ingredients:

- 2 tablespoons butter, melted and cooled
- 2 large organic eggs
- 2 ounces cream cheese, softened
- ¼ cup powdered Erythritol
- 1½ teaspoons organic vanilla extract
- Pinch of salt
- ¼ cup almond flour
- 2 tablespoons coconut flour
- 1 teaspoon organic baking powder

Directions:

Preheat a mini waffle iron and then grease it.

In a bowl, place the butter and eggs and beat until creamy.

Add the cream cheese, Erythritol, vanilla extract and salt and beat until well combined.

Add the flours and baking powder and beat until well combined.

Place ¼ of the mixture into preheated waffle iron and cook for about 4 minutes or until golden brown.

Repeat with the remaining mixture. Serve warm.

Nutrition Info:

Per Servings: Calories: 202 | Net Carb: 2. | Fat: 17.3g | Saturated Fat: 8g | Carbohydrates: 5.1g | Dietary Fiber: 2.3g| Sugar: 0.7g | Protein: 4.8g

Almond Butter Chaffles

Servings: 2

Cooking Time: 10 Minutes

Ingredients:

- 1 large organic egg, beaten
- 1/3 cup Mozzarella cheese, shredded
- 1 tablespoon Erythritol
- 2 tablespoons almond butter
- 1 teaspoon organic vanilla extract

Directions:

Preheat a mini waffle iron and then grease it.

In a medium bowl, place all ingredients and with a fork, mix until well combined.

Place half of the mixture into preheated waffle iron and cook for about 5 minutes or until golden brown.

Repeat with the remaining mixture.
Serve warm.

Nutrition Info:

Per Servings: Calories: 153 | Net Carb: 2g | Fat: 12.3g | Saturated Fat: 2g | Carbohydrates: 3. | Dietary Fiber: 1.6g | Sugar: 1.2g Protein: 7.9g

Pumpkin Chaffles

Servings: 2

Cooking Time: 12 Minutes

Ingredients:

- 1 organic egg, beaten
- ½ cup Mozzarella cheese, shredded
- 1½ tablespoon homemade pumpkin puree
- ½ teaspoon Erythritol
- ½ teaspoon organic vanilla extract
- ¼ teaspoon pumpkin pie spice

Directions:

Preheat a mini waffle iron and then grease it.

In a bowl, place all the ingredients and beat until well combined.

Place ¼ of the mixture into preheated waffle iron and cook for about 4-6 minutes or until golden brown.

Repeat with the remaining mixture.
Serve warm.

Nutrition Info:

Per Servings: Calories: 59 | Net Carb: 1.2g | Fat: 3.5g | Saturated Fat: 1.5g | Carbohydrates: 1. | Dietary Fiber: 0.4g | Sugar: 0.7g Protein: 4.9g

Churro Waffles

Servings: 1

Cooking Time: 10 Minutes

Ingredients:

- 1 tbsp coconut cream
- 1 egg
- 6 tbsp almond flour
- ¼ tsp xanthan gum
- ½ tsp cinnamon
- 2 tbsp keto brown sugar
- Coating:
- 2 tbsp butter, melt
- 1 tbsp keto brown sugar
- Warm up your waffle maker.

Directions:

Pour half of the batter to the waffle pan and cook for 5 minutes. Carefully remove the cooked waffle and repeat the steps with the remaining batter.
Allow the chaffles to cool and spread with the melted butter and top with the brown sugar.
Enjoy.

Nutrition Info:

Calories Per Servings: 178 Kcal | Fats: 15.7 g | Carbs: 3.9 g | Protein: 2 g

Oreo Chaffles

Servings: 2

Cooking Time: 5 Minutes

Ingredients:

- Chocolate Chaffle:
- 2 eggs
- 2 tbsp cocoa, unsweetened
- 2 tbsp sweetener
- 2 tbsp heavy cream
- 2 tsp coconut flour
- 1/2 tsp baking powder
- 1 tsp vanilla
- Filling:
- Whipped cream

Directions:

Pour half of the mixture into the waffle iron. Cook for 5 min- utes.

Once ready, carefully remove and repeat with the remaining chaffle mixture.

Allow the cooked chaffles to sit for 3 minutes.

Once they have cooled, spread the whipped cream on the chaf- fles and stack them cream side facing down to form a sandwich.

Slice into halves and enjoy.

Nutrition Info:

Calories Per Servings: 390 Kcal |Fats: 40 g | Carbs: 3 g

Protein: 10 g

Ube Chaffles With Ice Cream

Servings: 2

Cooking Time: 10 Minutes

Ingredients:

- 1/3 cup mozzarella cheese, shredded
- 1 tbsp whipped cream cheese
- 2 tbsp sweetener
- 1 egg
- 2-3 drops ube or pandan extract
- 1/2 tsp baking powder
- Keto ice cream

Directions:

Add in 2 or 3 drops of ube extract, mix until creamy and smooth.
Pour half of the batter mixture in the mini waffle maker and cook for about 5 minutes.
Repeat the same steps with the remaining batter mixture.
Top with keto ice cream and enjoy.
Note: more keto stuffing you can find in my easy desserts' cookbook here:

Nutrition Info:

Calories Per Servings:

265Kcal | Fats: 16 g | Carbs: 7 g | Protein: 22 g

Almond Flour Chaffles

Servings: 2

Cooking Time: 20 Minutes

Ingredients:

- 1 large egg
- 1 Tbsp blanched almond flour
- ¼ tsp baking powder
- ½ cup shredded mozzarella cheese

Directions:

Whisk egg, almond flour, and baking powder together.
Stir in mozzarella and set batter aside.

Turn on waffle maker to heat and oil it with cooking spray.

Pour half of the batter onto waffle maker and spread it evenly with a spoon.

Cook for 3 minutes, or until it reaches desired doneness. Transfer to a plate and repeat with remaining batter.

Let chaffles cool for 2-3 minutes to crisp up.

Nutrition Info:

Carbs: 2 g | Fat: 13 g | Protein: 10 g | Calories: 131

Gingerbread Chaffle

Servings: 2

Cooking Time: 5 Minutes

Ingredients:

- ½ cup mozzarella cheese grated
- 1 medium egg
- ½ tsp baking powder
- 1 tsp erythritol powdered
- ½ tsp ground ginger
- ¼ tsp ground nutmeg
- ½ tsp ground cinnamon
- ⅛ tsp ground cloves
- 2 Tbsp almond flour
- 1 cup heavy whipped cream
- ¼ cup keto-friendly maple syrup

Directions:

Turn on waffle maker to heat and oil it with cooking spray.
Beat egg in a bowl.

Add flour, mozzarella, spices, baking powder, and erythritol. Mix well. Spoon one half of the batter into waffle maker and spread out evenly. Close and cook for minutes.

Remove cooked chaffle and repeat with remaining batter.
Serve with whipped cream and maple syrup.

Nutrition Info:

Carbs: 5 g | Fat: 15 g | Protein: 12 g | Calories: 103

Chocolate Cherry Chaffles

Servings: 1

Cooking Time: 5 Minutes

Ingredients:

- 1 Tbsp almond flour
- 1 Tbsp cocoa powder
- 1 Tbsp sugar free sweetener
- ½ tsp baking powder
- 1 whole egg
- ½ cup mozzarella cheese shredded
- 2 Tbsp heavy whipping cream whipped
- 2 Tbsp sugar free cherry pie filling
- 1 Tbsp chocolate chips

Directions:

Turn on waffle maker to heat and oil it with cooking spray. Mix all dry components in a bowl.

Add egg and mix well. Add cheese and stir again.

Spoon batter into waffle maker and close. Cook for 5 minutes, until done.

Top with whipping cream, cherries, and chocolate chips.

Nutrition Info:

Carbs: 6 g | Fat: 1 g | Protein: 1 g | Calories: 130

Cinnamon Sugar Chaffles

Servings: 2

Cooking Time: 12 Minutes

Ingredients:

- 2 eggs
- 1 cup Mozzarella cheese, shredded
- 2 tbsp blanched almond flour
- ½ tbsp butter, melted
- 2 tbsp Erythritol
- ½ tsp cinnamon
- ½ tsp vanilla extract
- ½ tsp psyllium husk powder, optional
- ¼ tsp baking powder, optional
- 1 tbsp melted butter, for topping
- ¼ cup Erythritol, for topping
- ¾ tsp cinnamon, for topping

Directions:

Pour enough batter into the waffle maker and cook for 4 minutes.
Once the cooked, carefully remove the chaffle and set aside.
Repeat with the remaining batter the same steps.
Stir together the cinnamon and erythritol.
Finish by brushing your chaffles with the melted butter and then
sprinkle with cinnamon sugar.

Nutrition Info:

Calories Per Servings:

208 Kcal | Fats: 16 g | Carbs: 4 g | Protein: 11 g

Chocolate Chips & Whipping Cream Chaffles

Servings: 2

Cooking Time: 8 Minutes

Ingredients:

- 1 organic egg
- 1 tablespoon heavy whipping cream
- ½ teaspoon coconut flour
- 1¾ teaspoons monkfruit sweetener
- ¼ teaspoon organic baking powder
- Pinch of salt
- 1 tablespoon 70% dark chocolate chips

Directions:

Preheat a mini waffle iron and then grease it.

In a bowl, place all ingredients except for chocolate chips and beat until well combined.

Fold in the blackberries.

Place half of the mixture into preheated waffle iron and top with half of the chocolate chips.

Cook for about 3-4 minutes or until golden brown.
Repeat with the remaining mixture and chocolate chips.
Serve warm.

Nutrition Info:

Per Servings: Calories: 110 | Net Carb: 1. | Fat: 9g | Saturated Fat: 5g | Carbohydrates: 3.1g | Dietary Fiber: 1.3g | Sugar: 0.2g | Protein: 4g

Berries Chaffles

Servings: 2

Cooking Time: 10 Minutes

Ingredients:

- 1 organic egg
- 1 teaspoon organic vanilla extract
- 1 tablespoon of almond flour
- 1 teaspoon organic baking powder
- Pinch of ground cinnamon
- 1 cup Mozzarella cheese, shredded
- 2 tablespoons fresh blueberries
- 2 tablespoons fresh blackberries

Directions:

Preheat a waffle iron and then grease it.

In a bowl, place thee egg and vanilla extract and beat well. Add the flour, baking powder and cinnamon and mix well. Add the Mozzarella cheese and mix until just combined. Gently, fold in the berries.

Place half of the mixture into preheated waffle iron and cook for about 4-5 minutes or until golden brown.

Repeat with the remaining mixture.
Serve warm.

Nutrition Info:

Per Servings: Calories: 112 | Net Carb: 3.8g | Fat: 6.7g Saturated Fat: 2.3g | Carbohydrates: 5g | Dietary Fiber: 1.2g | Sugar: 1. Protein: 7g

Carrot Chaffles

Servings: 6

Cooking Time: 18 Minutes

Ingredients:

- ¾ cup almond flour
- 1 tablespoon walnuts, chopped
- 2 tablespoons powdered Erythritol
- 1 teaspoon organic baking powder
- ½ teaspoon ground cinnamon
- ½ teaspoon pumpkin pie spice
- 1 organic egg, beaten
- 2 tablespoons heavy whipping cream
- 2 tablespoons butter, melted
- ½ cup carrot, peeled and shredded

Directions:

Preheat a mini waffle iron and then grease it.

In a bowl, place the flour, walnut, Erythritol, cinnamon, baking powder and spices and mix well.

Add the egg, heavy whipping cream and butter and mix until well combined.

Gently, fold in the carrot.

Add about 3 tablespoons of the mixture into preheated waffle iron and cook for about 2½-3 minutes or until golden brown.

Repeat with the remaining mixture.
Serve warm.

Nutrition Info:

Per Servings: Calories: 165 | Net Carb: 2.4g | Fat: 14.7g | Saturated Fat: 4.4g | Carbohydrates: 4.4g | Dietary Fiber: 2g | Sugar: 1g Protein: 1.5g

Mocha Chaffles

Servings: 3

Cooking Time: 9 Minutes

Ingredients:

- 1 organic egg, beaten
- 1 tablespoon cacao powder
- 1 tablespoon Erythritol
- ¼ teaspoon organic baking powder
- 2 tablespoons cream cheese, softened
- 1 tablespoon mayonnaise
- ¼ teaspoon instant coffee powder
- Pinch of salt
- 1 teaspoon organic vanilla extract

Directions:

Preheat a mini waffle iron and then grease it.

In a medium bowl, place all ingredients and with a fork, mix until well combined.

Place 1/of the mixture into preheated waffle iron and cook for about 2½-3 minutes or until golden brown.

Repeat with the remaining mixture. Serve warm.

Nutrition Info:

Per Servings: Calories: 83 | Net Carb: 1g | Fat: 7.5g | Saturated Fat: 4. | Carbohydrates: 1.5g | Dietary Fiber: 0.5g | Sugar: 0.3g | Protein: 2.7g

Chocolate Vanilla Chaffles

Servings: 2

Cooking Time: 5 Minutes

Ingredients:

- ½ cup shredded mozzarella cheese
- 1 egg
- 1 Tbsp granulated sweetener
- 1 tsp vanilla extract
- 1 Tbsp sugar-free chocolate chips
- 2 Tbsp almond meal/flour

Directions:

Turn on waffle maker to heat and oil it with cooking spray. Mix all components in a bowl until combined.

Pour half of the batter into waffle maker.

Cook for 2-minutes, then remove and repeat with remaining batter. Top with more chips and favourite toppings.

Nutrition Info:

Carbs: 23 g | Fat: 3 g | Protein: 4 g | Calories: 134

CPSIA information can be obtained
at www.ICGtesting.com
Printed in the USA
BVHW092224040521
606416BV00009B/1161